# FIT FOR LIFE

## A COMPREHENSIVE GUIDE TO FITNESS AND WELLNESS

## A.D RAMS

# Contents

## CHAPTER ONE

## INTRODUCTION

This book is your reliable companion on the way to achieving and maintaining a lifestyle of fitness, wellness, and general well-being in a world where the pursuit of health and vitality is a lifelong journey. Welcome to "Fit for Life: A Comprehensive Guide to Fitness and Wellness."

It is impossible to emphasize how important it is to put our physical and mental health first in today's hectic culture. "Fit for Life" is intended to give you the information, resources, and motivation you need to start a life-changing path toward maximum health and vitality. Regardless of your level of experience with fitness or wellbeing, this book provides useful guidance, research-backed tactics, and doable actions to support you in achieving your objectives and leading the best possible life.

You'll find a plethora of knowledge on a variety of subjects in "Fit for Life," such as nutrition, stress management, exercise science, sleep hygiene, and more. Every chapter offers information, advice, and ideas to help you take charge of your health and flourish in all facets of your life, from creating efficient exercise regimens to choosing wholesome foods and developing an optimistic outlook.

"Fit for Life" is a holistic approach to wellbeing that acknowledges the connection between the mind, body, and spirit, but it's more than simply a manual. Through a thorough examination of the mental, emotional, and social aspects of health, this book provides a thorough framework for attaining resilience, vitality, and balance in an ever-more complicated environment.

Upon starting "Fit for Life," I encourage you to approach every chapter with an open mind, a curious attitude, and a dedication to self-discovery. Seize the chance to learn new things, disprove outdated notions, and develop wholesome behaviors that will benefit your long-term pleasure and health.

Recall that achieving fitness and wellness is a lifelong journey that calls for commitment, tenacity, and an openness to change rather than a destination. Together, let's set out on this road to achieve our common goals of wellbeing, contentment, and a life well lived.

Cheers to your well-being, energy, and the journey that lies ahead. Greetings from "Fit for Life."

## Fitness's Role in General Health and Well-Being

Fitness is essential to our general health and wellbeing since it affects not just our physical state but also our mental, emotional, and social well-being. For our overall well-being, fitness is essential for the following reasons:

Physical Health: Frequent exercise helps healthy weight management, increases muscular strength and endurance, and strengthens the cardiovascular system. It also improves flexibility. It helps people live longer and in better health by lowering their chance of developing chronic illnesses like diabetes, heart disease, obesity, and some types of cancer.

Mental Health: Exercise has a significant positive impact on mental health by reducing stress, anxiety, and depressive symptoms. Exercise lowers cortisol levels, the stress hormone, and increases the production of endorphins, neurotransmitters that enhance emotions of happiness and wellbeing. Frequent exercise also enhances memory, cognitive function, and general brain health.

Emotional Well-Being: Physical activity offers a way to release tension and express emotions, which helps to control mood and strengthen emotional resilience. Exercise increases self-esteem and promotes a good self-image by encouraging a sense of success and self-confidence.

Social Connection: Engaging in fitness activities provides chances for companionship, cooperation, and social interaction—all of which are critical for establishing a feeling of community and belonging. Activities like team sports, outdoor pursuits, and group fitness classes offer opportunities to meet new people, develop social support systems, and improve interpersonal ties.

Quality of Life: Having good physical health makes it easier and more efficient for us to carry out our everyday tasks, which raises our quality of life in general. It gives us more energy, lessens exhaustion, and encourages better sleep, which enables us to be more productive and lively every day.

Exercise is linked to a decreased risk of age-related decline and impairment, which helps people keep their independence and functional mobility as they age. This link explains the relationship between longevity and aging. Engaging in physical activity helps older persons maintain healthy bones, flexible joints, and a healthy muscle mass, which lowers their risk of fractures and falls.

Disease Prevention and Management: Exercise is essential for both avoiding and treating a number of illnesses, such as metabolic syndrome, osteoporosis, hypertension, and arthritis. Exercise boosts the body's capacity to fend against infections and inflammation, strengthens the immune system, and increases blood circulation.

Stress Management: Engaging in physical activity helps to naturally release tension, enhance relaxation, and foster mental clarity. People can relieve stored-up tension and find equilibrium and balance by exercising, which offers a healthy outlet for pent-up energy and emotions.

Ultimately, being fit is about nourishing our physical, mental, and emotional well-being and experiencing life to the fullest it has nothing to do with looking nice or developing a certain physique. We may improve our general health, happiness, and longevity by making regular exercise and physical activity a priority. This will enable us to thrive in all facets of our lives.

## Individual Relationship with Fitness

My relationship with exercise is deeply ingrained in my life, influencing many facets of it and helping me on my path to overall wellbeing. I learned early on about the significant effects physical activity had on my body and mind, as well as its transformational capacity.

I used to love being active as a kid whether it was dancing to my favorite music, playing sports with friends, or exploring the outdoors. These encounters gave me a passion for exercise and established the groundwork for a lifetime of fitness dedication.

Fitness evolved from a pastime during my teens and into adulthood to a haven, a source of strength, and a means of achieving self-discovery. Exercise gave me a sense of stability and control in stressful or uncertain times, enabling me to channel my energy constructively and find solace from life's obstacles.

I can personally attest to the positive physical advantages of consistent exercise. I've experienced the thrill of pushing myself to the edge during strenuous exercises, the fulfillment of setting new personal records, and the empowerment that results from taking charge of my fitness and well-being.

The advantages of fitness for the mind and emotions, however, can be much more significant. I've gained important knowledge about tenacity, resiliency, and self-control from exercising. I've come to understand the value of mindfulness and present, and I take comfort in the cadence of my breathing and my footsteps hitting the pavement.

For me, fitness has also been a means of community and connection. Whether it's through outdoor trips, recreational sports leagues, or group fitness courses, I've had the honor of developing deep connections with people who share my enthusiasm for health and wellness.

Above all, I am personally connected to fitness because I am grateful for the gift of movement, the chance to push myself, and the overall great sense of well-being it provides. Through it all, fitness has been a constant companion—a source of joy, inspiration, and vigor that enhances every aspect of my life. The path has been full of highs and lows, wins and disappointments.

## An overview of the goals and organization of the book

The goal of the book "Fit for Life: A Comprehensive Guide to Fitness and Wellness" is to empower readers as they travel toward reaching their ideal state of health and wellbeing. Its goal is to offer a comprehensive approach to fitness that takes into account one's social, mental, emotional, and physical well-being. This book seeks to direct readers toward a lifestyle that supports resilience, vitality, and longevity by providing useful guidance, evidence-based tactics, and doable actions.

"Fit for Life" is organized in an approachable manner and starts off by outlining the significance of wellbeing and exercise in our lives. The text delves into the interdependence of the mind, body, and spirit, highlighting the importance of promoting our overall health in order to lead a well-rounded and satisfying life.

After that, the book explores several aspects of health and fitness, including exercise science, diet, stress reduction, good sleep hygiene, and more. In-depth analyses, professional guidance, and helpful hints are included in every chapter to assist readers in incorporating fitness into their everyday life and overcoming typical obstacles they could run into.

## Recognizing Fitness

Comprehending fitness entails realizing the complex nature of physical health and the different elements that go into general well-being. The definition of fitness is broken down as follows:

Physical Fitness Components: Cardiovascular endurance, muscular strength, muscular endurance, flexibility, and body composition are some of the essential elements that make up fitness. Having a thorough understanding of these elements enables people to create comprehensive exercise programs that target various facets of physical health.

The ability of the heart, lungs, and blood arteries to supply oxygen to the body's tissues during an extended period of physical exercise is known as cardiovascular endurance. Cardiovascular endurance can be enhanced by engaging in exercises such brisk walking, cycling, swimming, and running.

The force that a muscle or group of muscles can produce in the face of resistance is referred to as muscular strength. Muscular strength can be effectively developed by strength training activities like bodyweight exercises, resistance band workouts, and weightlifting.

The capacity of a muscle or group of muscles to sustain repetitive contractions for a prolonged amount of time is known as muscular endurance. Muscular endurance is enhanced by low-resistance, high-repetition activities like bodyweight exercises and circuit training.

Flexibility: The range of motion at a joint or set of joints is referred to as flexibility. Pilates, yoga, and stretching techniques are good for preserving joint mobility and increasing flexibility.

Body Composition: The percentage of bone, muscle, fat, and other tissues in the body is referred to as body composition.

## CHAPTER TWO

Maintaining a balance between lean muscle mass and body fat through a combination of regular exercise and a healthy diet is necessary to achieve a healthy body composition.

Functional Fitness: Exercises that enhance movement patterns, balance, coordination, and stability are the main focus of functional fitness in addition to the conventional components of fitness. Functional exercises help people carry out daily tasks more easily and effectively by simulating real-life movements.

Progressive Overload: Reaching fitness objectives requires an understanding of the progressive overload theory. For the purpose of continuously challenging the body and encouraging adaptation and improvement, progressive overload refers to progressively increasing the intensity, duration, or frequency of exercise.

Rest and Recuperation: These are essential elements of every exercise regimen. Resting enough enables the body to rebuild and repair tissues, restore energy reserves, and adjust to the strain of exercise, which enhances performance and lowers the chance of injury.

Individualization: It's critical to understand that achieving fitness is a very personalized process. It's important to pay attention to your body, make reasonable goals, and customize your exercise regimen to suit your own needs, tastes, and skill level because what works for one person might not work for another.

Individuals can create thorough and efficient exercise regimens that support optimum health, strength, endurance, flexibility, and general well-being by comprehending these fundamental concepts of fitness.

## Creating Fitness Objectives

Establishing fitness objectives is a crucial first step in designing a disciplined and successful exercise program that fits your goals and incentives. This is a how-to for creating fitness objectives:

Establish Your Goals: To begin, make sure you know exactly what you hope to accomplish from your fitness adventure. Do you want to become more physically active, reduce weight, gain muscle, strengthen your heart, become more flexible, improve your athletic performance, or just live a healthier lifestyle? Setting goals will be guided by your understanding of your objectives.

Make Them specified: Establish time-bound, relevant, measurable, attainable, and specified

(SMART) goals. Rather than just stating, "I want to get fit," be more specific about your goals and a deadline. For instance, "I want to lose 10 pounds in three months," as well as "I want to be able to run a 5K race in six months."

Divide Them: Divide more ambitious objectives into more doable benchmarks. This helps you track your progress more efficiently and lessens the overwhelming nature of your goals. If your ultimate objective is to run a marathon, for instance, your benchmarks might be finishing a 5K race, finishing a half marathon, and progressively increasing your mileage over time.

Examine Various Fitness Domains: Examine the many fitness domains, including physical strength, flexibility, cardiovascular endurance, and body composition. To establish a comprehensive fitness plan, set goals that touch on all of these areas.

Have Reasonable Expectations: Be truthful with yourself about your existing level of fitness, your lifestyle, and any potential roadblocks you might run into. Establish goals that are difficult but doable, keeping in mind your unique situation and constraints.

Write Them Down: Whether it's in a fitness app, a notepad, or a whiteboard, put your goals down in writing. Setting down your objectives helps you be more accountable for them and gives them a more real, solid sense.

After your goals have been determined, make a detailed action plan that outlines the activities you must take to reach them. This could entail planning meals, scheduling exercise, getting advice from a specialist, and building rest and recuperation into your daily schedule.

Remain Adaptable: Allow yourself to make necessary modifications to your plan of action and goals in response to your physical progress, evolving situations, and feedback from your body. Being flexible enables you to continue on your fitness journey while embracing setbacks and celebrating victories.

Track Your Progress: Keep a close eye on how you're doing as you work toward your objectives, and acknowledge your successes along the way.

Maintaining a record of your exercises, measurements, and other pertinent information keeps you accountable and motivated while giving you insightful feedback on what's working and what needs to be changed.

Last but not least, maintain your commitment to your objectives in the face of obstacles or disappointments. Remain optimistic, concentrate on your advancement rather than perfection, and keep in mind that every step you take toward your ultimate fitness goals, no matter how tiny, will get you closer to your destination.

Establishing measurable, attainable, and purposeful exercise objectives will help you make a plan for success and start along a fulfilling path to better health, energy, and overall wellbeing.

## Elements of Health

Each of the many essential elements that make up fitness adds to one's overall physical health and wellbeing. By having a thorough understanding of these elements, people may create well-rounded exercise programs and successfully meet their fitness objectives. The primary elements of fitness are as follows:

Cardiovascular Endurance: The capacity of the heart, lungs, and circulatory system to supply oxygen-rich blood to working muscles over an extended period of physical exercise is referred to as cardiovascular endurance, also known as aerobic fitness. Exercises like cycling, swimming, jogging, dancing, and cycling all increase cardiovascular endurance.

The amount of force a muscle or group of muscles can apply against resistance in a single, peak effort is known as muscular strength. Exercises for building muscle strength and power include resistance band workouts, bodyweight exercises, and weightlifting.

The capacity of a muscle or group of muscles to sustain repeated contractions for a prolonged amount of time without experiencing tiredness is known as muscular endurance. Bodyweight exercises, circuit training, and high-repetition weightlifting are examples of endurance exercises that combine low resistance and high repetitions.

Flexibility: The range of motion at a joint or set of joints is referred to as flexibility. Stretching, yoga, Pilates, and mobility drills all help to increase muscle suppleness, joint mobility, and flexibility, which lowers the risk of injury and improves the quality of movement overall.

Body Composition: The percentage of bone, muscle, fat, and other tissues in the body is referred to as body composition. Maintaining a balance between lean muscle mass and body fat through a mix of regular exercise, a nutritious diet, and lifestyle choices is necessary to achieve a good body composition.

The capacity to keep control of the body's center of mass over its support system is known as balance. Exercises for balance test the body's proprioception, coordination, and stability. They also aid with posture, fall prevention, and performance enhancement in sports.

Coordination: The capacity to smoothly and effectively synchronize the actions of various bodily parts is known as coordination. Agility exercises, training tailored to a particular activity, and activities requiring fine motor skills, like dancing and martial arts, are all good ways to enhance coordination.

Agility is the capacity to alter course fast and effectively while retaining equilibrium and control. Exercises that improve agility include quick direction changes, acceleration, deceleration, and response to outside stimuli. They also lower the risk of injury while improving athletic performance.

Speed is the capacity to move rapidly between locations or to complete a task in a little period of time. The main goals of speed training exercises are to increase stride length and frequency, strengthen fast-twitch muscle fibers, and improve reaction time.

Power is the capacity to apply force rapidly by fusing speed and strength. Power is developed via plyometric workouts, Olympic lifting, and explosive activities like medicine ball tosses, sprints, and jumps. This improves functional ability and athletic performance.

An all-encompassing and balanced approach to physical health and performance can be attained by individuals by combining a range of exercises and activities that focus on various components of fitness. Taking care of each aspect of fitness whether your objective is to increase flexibility, increase strength and muscle, improve cardiovascular health, or perform better in sports and other activities will benefit your success and general well-being.

## Exercise for the Heart

Cardiovascular exercise, sometimes referred to as aerobic or cardio exercise, is a kind of exercise that works the heart and breathing muscles in order to develop cardiovascular fitness. It entails rhythmic, repetitive motions that work big muscles and increase oxygen uptake in the body. There are several advantages of cardiovascular exercise for general health and wellbeing, such as:

Better Heart Health: Engaging in cardiovascular exercise reduces the risk of heart disease, stroke, and high blood pressure by strengthening the heart muscle, increasing cardiac output, and improving circulation.

Improved Respiratory Function: Consistent cardiac activity increases lung volume and effectiveness, which increases the body's ability to absorb oxygen and expel carbon dioxide. Better respiratory health and greater physical activity endurance result from this.

Enhanced Energy: Cardiovascular activity increases energy levels through improved oxygen transport to tissues and enhanced metabolic efficiency. Frequent aerobic exercise can improve emotions of energy and wellbeing, decrease weariness, and increase stamina.

Weight management: Cardiovascular activity is a useful strategy for weight loss and weight management since it burns calories and contributes to the creation of a calorie deficit. Frequent cardiovascular exercise can assist people in achieving and maintaining a healthy body weight when paired with a balanced diet.

Better Mental and Mood: Engaging in cardiovascular activity releases endorphins, which are neurotransmitters that encourage happiness and well-being while lowering stress, anxiety, and depressive symptoms. Moreover, it increases the synthesis of dopamine and serotonin, two neurotransmitters linked to emotional equilibrium and mood control.

Improved Cognitive Function: Studies have indicated that regular cardiovascular exercise enhances memory, attention, and executive function. It encourages neuroplasticity, which is the brain's capacity to change and restructure in response to external stimuli, improving cognitive function and brain health.

Reduced Risk of Chronic Disease: Regular cardiovascular exercise can help reduce the chance of acquiring long-term conditions like type 2 diabetes, obesity, and some cancers. It helps prevent and treat diseases generally by lowering blood sugar, reducing inflammation, and improving insulin sensitivity.

Cardiovascular exercise examples include:

sprinting

cyclizing

Swimming

brisk strolling

Rope jumping

Dancing

Pulling a row

Kickboxing

classes that are aerobic

Aim for at least 150 minutes of moderate-intensity aerobic activity or 75 minutes of vigorous-intensity aerobic activity each week, together with muscle-strengthening activities on two or more days per week, to experience the advantages of cardiovascular exercise. Cardiovascular exercise is crucial for boosting general health, fitness, and well-being, regardless of your preference for steady-state cardio, high-intensity interval training (HIIT), or leisure activities like hiking or sports.

## Strengthening Exercise

Strength training, sometimes referred to as weight training or resistance training, is a type of exercise that builds and strengthens muscles using resistance. It entails utilizing the body's own weight, resistance bands, weight machines, or free weights to execute workouts that target particular muscle areas against resistance. Numerous advantages of strength training for general health, fitness, and functional ability include:

Increased Muscle Strength: By inflicting tiny damage to muscle fibers, which the body repairs and grows stronger over the course of recuperation, strength training increases muscle growth and strength. Muscular strength and power can be significantly increased over time with regular strength exercise.

Better Muscle Tone and Definition: Consistent strength training improves body composition by reducing body fat percentage and increasing muscle mass. This leads to better overall muscle tone and definition. It sculpts and forms the body, making it appear slimmer and more athletic.

Enhanced Metabolic Rate: By building muscle, which burns more calories at rest than fat, strength training increases metabolism. As a result, weight management and fat loss objectives are supported by a higher resting metabolic rate (RMR) and increased calorie expenditure throughout the day.

Improved Bone Health: Strength exercise, particularly for older persons, lowers the risk of osteoporosis and fractures by stimulating bone growth and increasing bone density. Weight-bearing activities that preserve bone strength and integrity include lunges, squats, and resistance training.

Strengthening the muscles around joints improves joint health and function by lowering the chance of injury and offering stability and support.

## CHAPTER THREE

Additionally, it increases range of motion, flexibility, and general joint health, which boosts mobility and functional ability.

Enhanced Sports Performance: For athletes and anyone taking part in physical activities and sports, strength training is crucial. It raises muscle power, strength, endurance, speed, and agility, which enhances athletic performance and lowers the chance of sports-related injuries.

Decreased Risk of Chronic Illness: Studies have indicated that strength training can reduce the incidence of long-term conditions such type 2 diabetes, heart disease, and arthritis. It enhances blood lipid profiles, cardiovascular health, and insulin sensitivity, which helps prevent and control diseases overall.

Enhanced Functional Capacity: Strength training increases mobility and functional strength, which facilitates daily tasks and lowers the risk of falls and injuries, particularly in older persons. It improves stability, balance, and coordination, which fosters independence and a higher standard of living.



Squats

Deadlifting

Bench Presses

Chin-ups and pull-ups

Lunges

Curls on the biceps

Dips of the triceps

Presses on the shoulders

Aim to complete resistance exercises for all major muscle groups two or three times a week, with enough time for rest and recuperation in between, in order to maximize the benefits of strength training. Over time, progressively raise the volume, resistance, and intensity of your workouts to keep pushing your muscles and encouraging growth. Strength training is a vital component of any fitness regimen, regardless of expertise level, as it helps improve body composition, increase strength, and improve general health and well-being.

## Adaptability and Mobility

Essential elements of physical fitness that support general health, wellbeing, and functional ability are flexibility and mobility. Although they are sometimes used synonymously, flexibility and mobility relate to a few distinct features of movement:

The ability of a muscle or group of muscles to extend passively through a range of motion is referred to as flexibility. It entails stretching connective tissues and muscles to release restrictions and enable joints to move easily and freely. Increased flexibility improves sports performance, lowers the chance of injury, and encourages better posture and movement mechanics.

On the other hand, mobility refers to the capacity to move a specific joint or group of joints through their full range of motion in an active and efficient manner. It includes joint stability, neuromuscular control, movement patterning, and muscle flexibility. Better balance, coordination, and agility are made possible by increased mobility, which benefits both daily tasks and sports performance.

## Advantages of Mobility and Flexibility:

Injury Prevention: By enhancing tissue resilience, lowering muscle imbalances, and improving joint mechanics, maintaining appropriate flexibility and mobility lowers the risk of musculoskeletal injuries. It aids in preventing sprains, strains, and other typical ailments brought on by exercise and day-to-day mobility.

Enhanced Performance: For the best possible athletic performance in sports and physical activities, flexibility and mobility are essential. They enable athletes to move more effectively, exert more energy and strength, and control and precisely carry out their activities. A stronger sense of suppleness also improves coordination, speed, and agility.

Enhanced Range of Motion: People can move more freely and easily when their flexibility and mobility combine to increase joint range of motion. Precise and unhindered movement in multiple planes of motion is possible with adequate flexibility and mobility, whether one is bending, twisting, reaching, or crouching.

Improved Posture: Maintaining appropriate posture and alignment throughout the body depends in large part on flexibility and mobility. They assist in mitigating the adverse impacts of extended periods of sitting, inactive lifestyles, and repeated motions, diminishing the likelihood of malpositions, taut muscles, and soreness.

Pain relief: Mobility and flexibility exercises can relieve chronic pain issues like neck, back, and joint stiffness by reducing muscular tension, stiffness, and discomfort. Frequent mobility exercises and stretches aid in the release of tense muscles, circulation, and the promotion of calmness and stress reduction.

Functional Movement: To carry out daily duties and activities with ease and efficiency, flexibility and mobility are necessary. Keeping one's flexibility and mobility at their best improves one's ability to perform functional movement patterns and quality of life, whether one is bending to pick up objects, reaching high, or crouching to sit and stand.

## Exercises to Improve Flexibility and Mobility:

Stretching in a static manner

Exertion in motion

Rolling foam

Yoga

Pilates

Drills for mobility

cooperative mobilizations

Exercises for range of motion, both active and passive

Regular flexibility and mobility exercise is crucial for preserving maximum physical performance, avoiding injuries, and enhancing general health and wellbeing. It should be a part of any fitness regimen. Stretching and mobility will help you achieve your long-term fitness objectives and improve your quality of life, whether you're an athlete trying to increase performance or a layperson aiming to reduce discomfort and improve movement quality.

## Energizing Your Exercise: Nutrition Before and After

It's essential to fuel your exercises with the right foods before and after to support recovery, maximize performance, and reach your fitness objectives. The following is a summary of pre- and post-exercise nutrition techniques to assist you maximize your fitness:

Before-Workout Diet:

Hydration: Drink plenty of water in the days before your workout to ensure that you are well hydrated. Try to drink 16–20 ounces of water two to three hours before working out, and another 8 10 ounces ten to twenty minutes before you begin.

Carbohydrates: To feed your muscles and provide you prolonged energy, eat a meal or snack high in carbohydrates one to three hours before exercising. Choose complex carbs that release glucose into the bloodstream gradually, such as those found in whole grains, fruits, vegetables, and legumes.

Protein: You can promote muscle growth and repair by including a small amount of protein in your pre-workout meal or snack. Select plant foods high in protein, such as beans and lentils, or lean protein sources, such as chicken, fish, tofu, and Greek yogurt.

Steer clear of foods high in fat and fiber: Although fiber and good fats are necessary for a balanced diet, they can impede digestion and make exercise uncomfortable. Steer clear of large, high-fat meals and foods high in fiber right before working out to avoid stomach problems.

Timing: To ensure optimal nutritional absorption and digestion, try to have your pre-workout meal or snack one to three hours before to doing out. Try different timings to see what suits your demands and the unique requirements of your body.

## After-Workout Nutrition:

Hydration: To restore fluids lost through perspiration, rehydrate your body after exercise by consuming water or a sports drink. Make sure you consume a minimum of 16-24 ounces of liquid for each pound of weight lost while exercising.

Carbohydrates: Eating carbohydrates restores glycogen stores and aids in the healing of muscles after exercise. To replenish your muscles, choose for high-quality, readily digested carbohydrates like whole grains, fruits, rice cakes, or sports drinks.

Protein: For muscle growth and repair, include protein in your post-workout meal or snack. To optimize the synthesis of muscle protein and promote recovery, try to eat a combination of carbohydrates and protein within 30 to 60 minutes of working out.

Timing of Nutrient Uptake: Often called the "anabolic window," the post-exercise period is crucial for muscle regeneration and nutrient absorption. During this time, eating a well-balanced meal or snack high in protein and carbs helps speed up recovery and encourage muscle adaption.

Protein Sources: For post-workout nutrition, choose quick-digesting protein sources such whey protein, eggs, Greek yogurt, or lean meats. Smoothies or protein drinks can also be practical choices for replenishing quickly and simply after a workout.

Recovery Snacks: A recovery snack might help you fill in the time until your next meal if you're not able to eat a full meal right after working out. A protein shake with fruit or yogurt with oats or a banana and peanut butter are good examples of a combination of carbs and protein.

Individual Needs: Modify your post-exercise nutrition according to your goals, the length and intensity of your workout, and any dietary preferences or constraints you may have. Try a variety of foods and timing techniques to see what suits you the best and advances your fitness objectives.

You can optimize your exercises, boost muscle recovery, maximize your performance, and move closer to your fitness goals by paying attention to your pre- and post-exercise diet and providing your body with the right nutrients at the right times.

## The Effects of Hydration on Fitness

Hydration affects a number of physiological processes necessary for the best possible physical activity, making it an important factor in fitness and exercise performance. Let's examine hydration and how it affects fitness in more detail:

## The Value of Hydration

Control of Body Temperature: The body produces heat when exercising, which raises the core temperature. By encouraging sweating and heat dissipation, enough hydration helps control body temperature and guards against overheating and heat-related ailments including heat exhaustion and heatstroke.

Preservation of Fluid Balance: Staying hydrated is crucial for preserving the body's fluid balance, which is vital for general health and wellbeing. The movement of nutrients and waste materials throughout the body, as well as the healthy operation of cells, tissues, and organs, depend on the right balance of bodily fluids.

Optimal Muscle Function: By guaranteeing sufficient blood flow and nutrient delivery to active muscles, hydration promotes optimal muscle function and performance. Dehydration can affect the strength, power, endurance, and contraction of muscles, which lowers exercise performance and raises the risk of injury.

Hydration aids in joint lubrication and cushioning, which lessens wear and friction when engaging in physical activity. Maintaining adequate hydration during exercise can help reduce joint pain, stiffness, and discomfort, enabling more fluid and comfortable movement.

Electrolyte equilibrium: Essential for fluid equilibrium, neuron function, muscular contraction, and other physiological functions are minerals including sodium, potassium, chloride, and magnesium. Electrolyte imbalances that might result from dehydration are avoided by drinking enough water to keep the body's electrolyte balance stable.

# CHAPTER FOUR

## Effect on Physical Fitness:

Exercise Performance: By promoting muscular, thermoregulatory, and cardiovascular health, optimal hydration improves exercise performance. Dehydration, even mildly, can affect one's ability to function, resulting in decreased strength, power, endurance, and coordination when engaging in physical exercise.

Endurance and stamina: Those who participate in extended or strenuous exercise, as well as endurance athletes, should pay special attention to maintaining adequate water. Dehydration can impair the ability to maintain exercise intensity and duration by causing tiredness, diminished stamina, and a decline in performance.

Recovery and Muscle healing: Hydration is essential for the restoration of lost fluids, the intake of nutrients, the healing of damaged muscles, and the resynthesis of glycogen after exercise. Maintaining adequate hydration speeds up the healing process between exercises by easing discomfort in the muscles.

Cognitive Function: During exercise, dehydration can affect one's ability to concentrate, pay attention, and make decisions, which can cause problems with focus, coordination, and reaction speed. Drinking enough of water during exercise promotes mental focus and alertness, which improves performance.

Injury Prevention: Staying properly hydrated lowers the chance of exercise-related ailments like strains and cramps in the muscles, as well as heat-related illnesses. Dehydration increases the risk of weariness, weakens joints, and impairs muscular function, all of which enhance an individual's vulnerability to injury during physical exercise.

## Guidelines for Hydration:

Pre-Exercise Hydration: To guarantee you're well hydrated before you begin your workout, consume water or a sports drink two to three hours beforehand.

Drink fluids frequently when exercising to replenish fluids lost through perspiration. Try to drink 7–10 ounces of fluid every 10–20 minutes, modifying your consumption according to the type, length, and intensity of your workout.

Post-Exercise Hydration: To replace lost fluid and aid in recovery, rehydrate after working out with water or a sports drink. Make sure you drink 16–24 ounces of fluid for each pound you lose while working out.

Keep an eye on your level of hydration. Look out for symptoms of dehydration, such as weariness, dizziness, dark urine, and thirst. It can be helpful to weigh oneself before and after exercise to determine your level of hydration and fluid loss.

Individual Needs: The amount of water required varies based on body size, type, intensity, length, and rate of perspiration during exercise. To suit your unique hydration demands, modify the amount of fluid you consume.

Hydration is essential for maximizing physical performance, promoting recovery, and lowering the risk of dehydration-related problems. It should be prioritized before, during, and after exercise. Maintaining optimal health and well-being as well as reaching your exercise objectives requires prioritizing hydration as part of your overall fitness program.

## Rest and Recuperation

Any fitness program must include recovery and rest since they are critical for maximizing results, avoiding injuries, and enhancing general wellbeing. Here's a closer look at how crucial rest and recuperation are to fitness:

## The Value of Healing

Muscle Growth and Repair: When you workout, your muscles break down and sustain microscopic damage. Over time, muscle growth and greater strength are attributed to the body's ability to repair and regenerate muscle tissues during recovery.

Reduction of Inflammation: The body may experience oxidative stress and inflammation as a result of intense physical activity. Sufficient recuperation mitigates inflammation, promoting tissue repair and lowering the chance of overuse injuries.

Restoring Energy Stores: After an activity session, the body can restore the glycogen stores that were lost. After a workout, consuming carbohydrates helps replenish energy in the muscles and prepare them for more exercise.

Hormonal Balance: Excessive exercise has the potential to upset the hormonal equilibrium, which raises levels of stress chemicals like cortisol. Restoring hormonal balance through enough rest and recuperation supports general health and wellbeing.

Preventing Overtraining: When the body experiences excessive physical stress without enough time for recovery, overtraining takes place. This may result in symptoms including exhaustion, irritation, and lowered immunity, as well as a decline in performance and an increased risk of injury.

## The Value of Rest

Muscle Recovery: After strenuous activity, muscles need time to rest and repair. This lowers the chance of damage while also encouraging the formation of new muscles and stronger muscles.

Recovery of the Central Nervous System: Excessive physical activity strains the central nervous system (CNS). Intervals of rest allow the central nervous system (CNS) to heal, resulting in enhanced motor function, response time, and general performance.

Mental and Emotional Health: Getting enough sleep is crucial for maintaining mental and emotional health. It offers time for unwinding, reducing stress, and recharging the mind, which helps to stave off burnout and enhance motivation and focus.

Sleep Quality: Getting enough sleep is crucial for general health and recuperation. The body repairs itself, regulates hormones, and consolidates memories while we sleep—all functions critical to health and performance.

Injury Prevention: By enabling the body to recuperate from physical strain and mend any damage sustained during activity, rest is essential for preventing injuries. Additionally, it aids in spotting and treating early indications of overuse or injury before they worsen.

## Techniques for Rest and Recuperation That Work:

Active Recovery: On days off, take part in low-impact, mild exercise like yoga, swimming, or walking to increase blood flow, lessen pain in your muscles, and accelerate healing.

Nutrition: To aid in healing and restock energy reserves, eat meals high in nutrients and drink enough of water. Make sure your post-workout meals and snacks contain healthy fats, protein, and carbohydrates.

Sleep: Make great sleep your top priority by adhering to a regular sleep schedule, furnishing a peaceful sleeping space, and adopting healthy sleeping practices.

Stress management: To encourage relaxation and mental health, include stress-reduction methods like deep breathing, meditation, or mindfulness exercises.

Listen to Your Body: Pay attention to the cues your body gives you, and modify the intensity, frequency, and length of your training sessions accordingly. Take breaks when necessary, and don't be afraid to take more days off if you're feeling exhausted or exhibiting overtraining symptoms.

You may improve performance, lower your chance of injury, and advance your long-term health and well-being by making rest and recovery a priority in your workout regimen. To support your fitness objectives and guarantee long-term, sustainable improvement, make sure your training plan includes enough rest and recuperation techniques.

## Including Mind-Body Techniques

Including mind-body techniques in your exercise regimen can boost performance, support holistic health, and increase general well-being. In order to promote balance, relaxation, and stress reduction, mind-body activities center on developing awareness, mindfulness, and a connection between the mind and body. The following well-liked mind-body exercises could be included in your exercise routine:

1. Yoga:

Benefits: Yoga encourages relaxation and relieves stress while enhancing flexibility, strength, balance, and posture. Additionally, it improves bodily awareness and mindfulness, which supports people in connecting with their inner selves and breathing.

Types: There are many different kinds of yoga, including as restorative, vinyasa, ashtanga, yin, and haiku. Select a look that complements your preferences and fitness objectives.

2. Pilates:

Advantages: Pilates emphasizes alignment, flexibility, stability, and core strength. In order to promote general body awareness and useful movement patterns, it places a strong emphasis on controlled movements, breath awareness, and the mind-body connection.

Types: Pilates can be done with specific equipment such a reformer, chair, or Cadillac, or it can be done on a mat. Pilates on a mat or with equipment has its own advantages and difficulties.

3. Tai Chi:

Benefits: Tai Chi is a gentle martial art that emphasizes deep breathing and slow, flowing movements. It elevates mental clarity, lowers tension, and enhances flexibility, balance, coordination, and relaxation.

Types: Tai Chi is a set of motions or forms that are executed continuously and fluidly. All fitness levels can practice it, and it can be done while sitting or standing.

4. Practice meditation:

Benefits of meditation include decreased tension, anxiety, and negative emotions as well as mindfulness, concentration, and relaxation. It raises one's level of self-awareness and encourages serenity and inner peace.

Types: There are many different kinds of meditation practices, such as body scan, loving-kindness, breath awareness, mindfulness, and guided meditation. Try out many methods until you find one that speaks to you.

5. Breathing exercises:

Benefits: The goal of breathwork is to reduce stress, increase emotional equilibrium, and promote relaxation through conscious breathing exercises. They relax the nervous system and improve energy, oxygenation, and mental clarity.

Types: Diaphragmatic breathing, box breathing (square breathing), and alternating nostril breathing (Nadi Shodhana) are a few examples of breathwork techniques. Investigate various methods to determine which ones best fit your requirements and tastes.

6. Moving With Awareness:

Benefits: Mindful movement techniques integrate physical movement with mindfulness and bodily awareness. Examples of these techniques include Feldenkrais, Qigong, and walking meditation. They encourage better mind-body awareness, relaxation, and a decrease in tension.

Types: Select mindful movement exercises that support your fitness objectives and speak to you personally. Try out a variety of modalities to see which ones are pleasurable and nourishing.

Including mind-body techniques in your exercise regimen can improve the effectiveness of your sessions overall, encourage stress relief and relaxation, and support holistic health and well-being. Whether you like the controlled motions of Tai Chi, the dynamic flow of yoga, or the precision of Pilates, choose practices that speak to you and incorporate them into your workout routine for a well-rounded and satisfying approach to health and fitness.

## Health Throughout Life

Every stage of life, from birth to old age, requires fitness. For people of all ages, establishing and maintaining a regular exercise regimen and physical activity levels can offer a multitude of advantages that enhance general health, wellbeing, and quality of life. Here is a look at fitness during the life course and how exercise can help each stage of health and vitality:

### Early Life (Ages 0–12):

Physical Development: Children who engage in regular physical activity benefit from improved motor abilities, coordination, and muscle strength. Healthy development and growth are encouraged by organized play and scheduled activities.

Cognitive Function: Research has demonstrated that physical activity improves children's attention span, academic achievement, and cognitive function. Exercise and active play promote learning and academic success by stimulating brain development.

Social Skills: Playing team sports and engaging in group activities helps kids develop their leadership, cooperation, teamwork, and social skills. Additionally, it fosters resilience, self-worth, and confidence.

## CHAPTER FIVE

### Teenage Years (Ages 13–19):

Physical Fitness: Adolescents who regularly exercise can develop stronger, more resilient muscles, and a better cardiovascular system. Engaging in sports and physical exercise encourages the development of healthy habits and lowers the chance of obesity and chronic illness in later life.

Mental Health: Research has demonstrated that physical activity helps teenagers feel less stressed, anxious, and depressed while also building resilience and emotional well-being. During this phase of change, exercise also improves happiness, self-worth, and body image and perception.

Healthy Habits: Forming lifetime health habits during adolescence is crucial. The basis for lifelong health and wellbeing is laid at this time by promoting frequent exercise and healthy lifestyle choices.

## Adulthood (20–64 Years Old):

Physical Health: Engaging in regular exercise as an adult contributes to the maintenance of bone density, muscle strength, flexibility, and cardiovascular health. By lowering the risk of chronic illnesses including diabetes, osteoporosis, and heart disease, it increases life expectancy and quality of life.

Weight Management: Exercise is essential for maintaining a healthy weight and lowering the risk of obesity-related disorders. It also plays a significant effect in body composition.

Stress Reduction: Engaging in physical activity is a great way for people to decompress and cope with the responsibilities of daily life, job, and family. Exercise raises mood, encourages relaxation, and strengthens mental health in general.

## Senior Adulthood (Persons 65 and Above):

Exercise in later life contributes to the maintenance of functional fitness, mobility, and independence. It boosts daily living activities, balance, and lowers the risk of falls.

Chronic Disease Management: For older persons, engaging in regular physical exercise can help manage chronic illnesses like osteoporosis, hypertension, and arthritis. It relieves pain, improves symptoms, and improves general health and quality of life.

Cognitive Health: Research has demonstrated that exercise helps older persons' cognitive performance and brain health, which lowers their risk of dementia and cognitive decline. It promotes cognitive vigor and well-being by improving memory, attention, and executive function.

## Important Things to Think About Throughout Life:

Individual Needs: People have varying fitness requirements and capacities depending on their stage of life. Exercise plans should be customized to each person's needs, preferences, and goals, taking into account things like mobility restrictions, fitness level, and health state.

Safety: At any age, put your safety first when exercising. To avoid injury, take it slow, warm up properly, and employ the right form and technique. Before beginning a new fitness regimen, speak with your doctor, particularly if you have any underlying medical issues.

Enjoyment: Pick pursuits that suit your interests and lifestyle while also being enjoyable. Whether it's dancing, yoga, cycling, swimming, or any other activity, find things to do that make you happy and include fitness into your life.

People can increase health, energy, and well-being at every age by integrating regular exercise and physical activity into their everyday lives. Fitness should be a top priority for everyone, regardless of age, as it is essential to a happy and healthy living.

## Overcoming Obstacles in the Fitness Domain

Establishing and sustaining a regular exercise regimen that promotes health and well-being requires overcoming obstacles to fitness. While individual barriers to physical activity may differ, many people encounter similar difficulties in their efforts to maintain an active lifestyle.

These are some methods for getting beyond obstacles in the way of fitness:

1. Insufficient Time:

Exercise should be prioritized, so plan it into your daily schedule just like you would any other significant commitment. Whether it's in the morning, during lunch, or in the evening, set out specific time for physical activity.

Divide It Up: If scheduling a long workout seems impossible, divide your workouts into shorter, more doable chunks spaced out throughout the day. Exercise for even ten to fifteen minutes each day can have a big impact on your health.

Combine Activities: Whenever possible, try to include physical activity into your other daily responsibilities. Use the stairs rather than the elevator, ride a bike or walk to work, or perform bodyweight exercises while watching television.

2. Absence of drive:

Make Goals: To stay motivated and engaged, make sure your exercise goals are clear and attainable. Whether your goal is to run a 5K, learn a new yoga posture, or gain more strength, having specific goals will motivate you to stick with your fitness regimen.

Select Pleasurable Activities: Opt for pursuits that you sincerely find enjoyable and eager to engage in. Whether it's hiking, dancing, athletics, or martial arts, engage in things that you enjoy to make working out feel more like an enjoyable activity than a chore.

Mix It Up: Try a variety of exercises and activities to keep your training fresh and engaging. To keep your body and mind active, change up your cardio, strength training, flexibility, and balancing routines.

3. Absence of Assistance:

Find a Workout Partner: Having a friend, relative, or coworker as a workout partner can offer social support, accountability, and incentive. Exercise can be more pleasurable and help you remain on track if you have a workout partner with whom to share your fitness journey.

Join a Group or exercise Class: Taking part in sports leagues or group exercise programs can foster a sense of community and togetherness. It can be motivating and supportive to be surrounded by people who have similar fitness aspirations.

Seek Professional Advice: To receive individualized advice, accountability, and motivation, it may be beneficial to collaborate with a personal trainer, fitness coach, or exercise physiologist. A specialist can assist you in developing a personalized fitness program and overcoming any difficulties you might run across.

4. Physical Restraints:

Speak with a Healthcare Professional: Before beginning a new fitness regimen, speak with a healthcare practitioner if you have any medical conditions or physical restrictions that limit your ability to exercise. Depending on your unique demands and health state, they can offer advice on safe and suitable activity.

Adapt workouts: Adjust workouts to your physical limits or ailments, and opt for low-impact, joint-friendly activities. Concentrate on tasks that you can complete with ease, then increase the difficulty as your fitness level rises.

Examine Other Exercise Options: Take into account other exercise options like chair yoga, tai chi, swimming, or water aerobics that might be more appropriate for your needs and skill level. These mild, low-impact exercises can minimize the chance of injury while still offering major health advantages.

5. Insufficient Resources:

Use Low-Cost or Free options: Make use of low-cost or free options for exercise, such as public parks or trails, walking or running in your neighborhood, or using fitness apps and online workout videos.

Exercise at Home: Set up a small exercise area in your home with basic tools like yoga mats, dumbbells, and resistance bands. Numerous efficient bodyweight workouts and exercises exist that need little to no equipment.

Investigate Community Resources: Look for community centers, neighborhood gyms, or leisure centers that provide group exercise programs, recreational sports leagues, or memberships at a reduced cost or on a sliding scale. For inhabitants, several municipalities also offer free or subsidized programs.

6. Emotional and Mental Barriers:

Develop self-compassion by treating yourself with kindness and accepting that failures and bad days are normal. Prioritize progress above perfection, and acknowledge and appreciate your accomplishments along the way.

Address Mental Health Needs: Consult a therapist or counselor for professional assistance if mental health conditions like anxiety, depression, or stress are interfering with your ability to exercise. Improving motivation and general wellbeing can be facilitated by addressing underlying mental health issues.

Incorporate Mind-Body Practices: To lower stress, promote relaxation, and sharpen your mind, incorporate mind-body activities like yoga, meditation, or deep breathing exercises into your daily routine. These techniques can aid in mental relaxation and foster an optimistic outlook on fitness.

7. Budgetary Obstacles:

Examine Inexpensive Options: Seek out low-cost fitness options including outdoor parks, community centers, or free internet workout videos. You may work out from home for free or at a reduced cost using a lot of fitness apps and websites.

Fees should be negotiated: If you're thinking about joining a gym or fitness center, find out about special offers for new customers, discounted rates for students or seniors, and flexible payment schedules. Depending on their income, some gyms may also charge sliding-scale prices.

Make Your Own Fitness: Use your imagination to come up with ways to work out without having to pay for pricey memberships or equipment. Exercises like walking, running, hiking, cycling, and bodyweight exercises are all inexpensive and beneficial kinds of physical activity.

Through proactive identification and resolution of fitness-related hurdles, you may surmount setbacks, maintain motivation, and create a long-lasting workout regimen that benefits your overall health and wellbeing. Keep in mind that development might not always be linear, and it's acceptable to ask for help and modify your strategy when necessary. You may overcome obstacles in your way of fitness and reach your health and fitness objectives with persistence, patience, and an optimistic outlook.

## Discovering Happiness in Motion

Establishing a fitness regimen that satisfies your body and soul while being sustainable and enjoyable requires you to find joy in exercise. Exercise turns from a chore into a source of empowerment and enjoyment when it becomes gratifying. The following are some methods for appreciating movement:

1. Examine Various Activities:

Try New Things: See what you enjoy most by trying out a range of sports and physical activities. Everyone can find something to enjoy, whether it's dancing, hiking, swimming, cycling, or martial arts.

Mix It Up: Use a variety of exercises and activities to keep your training captivating and exciting. To challenge your body and keep things interesting, alternate between aerobic, weight training, flexibility, and balancing activities.

2. Accept Playfulness:

Reach Out to Your Inner Child: Treat exercise with the same interest and playfulness that you did when you were younger. Move freely—jump, skip, hop without worrying about being judged or self-conscious.

Play Games: To make your workouts more enjoyable and engaging, turn them into games or challenges. Play tag, get your buddies together for a fun game of sports, or check out board games or applications that focus on fitness.

3. Discover Your Flow:

Focus on the Present: When working out, engage in mindfulness exercises and give your whole attention to the present. Let go of concerns and distractions while you focus on the exercise itself, your breath, and the feelings in your body.

Achieve a state of flow in which you are totally engrossed in the task at hand and lose sight of time. Experiences in flow are incredibly gratifying and fulfilling, bringing happiness and contentment.

4. Establish a Connection with Nature:

Get Outside: Exercise outside while taking in the scenery. Spending time in natural environments can improve your mood and strengthen your connection to movement, whether you're doing yoga in a park, going on a picturesque trek, or running by the shore.

Enjoy the Beauty: When you work out outside, take some time to enjoy the beauty of your surroundings. Take in the sights, sounds, and feelings of the natural world and allow it to enliven and inspire you.

5. Honor Your Advancement:

Concentrate on What You Can Do: Celebrate what your body is capable of doing instead of focusing on appearance or performance objectives. No matter where you are in your fitness path, acknowledge and appreciate your overall ability, strength, flexibility, and endurance.

Acknowledge Your Achievements: No matter how minor, acknowledge and celebrate your accomplishments. Take satisfaction in your achievements, whether it's finishing a difficult workout, setting a new personal record, or learning a new skill.

## 6. Talk About Your Experience:

Exercise with Friends: Ask loved ones to accompany you on your fitness adventures. It might be more fun and inspiring to exercise with others since it fosters social support and connection.

Join a Community: Take part in online communities dedicated to your favorite pastimes, sports leagues, or group fitness courses. Being surrounded by people who share your values might improve your satisfaction and sense of belonging.

7. Pay Attention to Your Body:

Respect Your Body: Be aware of your body's signals and be mindful of its requirements and constraints. Opt for energetic and pleasurable activities and intensities rather than pushing oneself to the brink of pain or discomfort.

Adjust as Necessary: Have an open mind and be prepared to change up your training regimen according to your current state of mind. If anything doesn't seem right, change activities, alter the intensity of the workouts, or both.

8. Develop Gratitude:

Feel Appreciation: Give thanks for being able to move your body and perform physical activities. Express gratitude for the strength, energy, and happiness that exercise provides to your life and recognize it as a priceless gift.

Consider the Benefits: Give some thought to the ways that exercising improves your emotional, mental, and physical health.

## CHAPTER SIX

Observe how getting more exercise improves your energy, elevates your mood, and makes life better overall.

Finding activities that truly speak to you and embracing the joy of movement will help you develop a lifelong connection with fitness that will bring you fulfillment, vitality, and happiness. Recall that exercise is about more than just losing weight or accomplishing objectives; it's also about taking care of your body, mind, and soul and appreciating life to the fullest.

## Monitoring Results and Modifying Objectives

Maintaining a successful and long-lasting fitness journey requires monitoring progress and making goal adjustments. You may stay motivated, keep up the momentum, and keep moving in the direction of your goals by keeping an eye on your accomplishments and making the required modifications along the road. The following techniques can be used to properly monitor progress and make goal adjustments:

1. Set Specific, Measurable Objectives:

Specificity: Make sure your goals are clear and precise, outlining your desired outcomes. Clarity is essential whether one is trying to gain strength, increase endurance, lose weight, or learn a new skill.

Measurability: Make sure your objectives can be measured so you can monitor your development over time. To quantify your success, use quantitative indicators like weight, body measurements, time, distance, repetitions, or performance benchmarks.

2. Select the Correct Tracking Techniques:

Keep a Journal: To document your exercises, advancements, and accomplishments, keep a journal or use a digital tracking tool. Add specifics like the kind of exercise, length, intensity, number of sets, repetitions, weights, and any other pertinent information.

Use Technology: Make use of wearables, smartphone apps, and fitness trackers that can measure your heart rate, steps taken, calories burned, and sleep quality, among other aspects of your fitness. These resources offer insightful information on your activity levels and development.

3. Track important performance metrics:

Frequent Assessments: Arrange for regular evaluations to gauge your fitness level and track your development. Utilize instruments like performance reviews, body composition assessments, and fitness testing to gauge progress and pinpoint areas that want work.

Track Trends: As your data accumulates, keep an eye out for patterns and trends. To get a complete picture of your development, track changes in energy, mood, body composition, performance, and general well-being.

4. Honor accomplishments and landmarks:

Celebrate your victories and accomplishments along the road, no matter how minor. Acknowledge your development, diligence, and commitment, and feel proud of your achievements.

Reward Yourself: Give yourself incentives or rewards when you accomplish important milestones or particular objectives. Discover strategies to acknowledge and maintain your motivation, such as treating yourself to a massage, a fun outing, or a new training attire.

5. Remain Adaptable and Flexible:

Be Open to Change: Keep an open mind and be prepared to modify your objectives in light of your development, personal preferences, and evolving circumstances. Acknowledge that objectives could change over time and be willing to make the necessary adjustments.

Listen to Your Body: Pay attention to the cues your body gives you, and modify the intensity, frequency, and length of your workout as necessary. Take breaks when needed, adjust your exercise regimen, or get help from a specialist if you run into problems or setbacks.

6. Make New Objectives and Challenges:

Continuous Growth: To stay motivated and interested in your work, set new challenges for yourself after you've reached a goal or milestone. Whether it's gaining weight, gaining speed, learning complex methods, or taking on new activities, push yourself to new limits.

Strike a balance between ambition and realism by setting high but manageable objectives that will challenge you without sacrificing your reach. Achieve a balance between pushing yourself and positioning yourself for achievement.

7. Seek Assistance and Responsibility:

Share Your Objectives: Let others who can provide accountability, inspiration, and support—friends, family, or a supportive community—know what your objectives are. Along your fitness journey, having a support system can help you stay accountable and inspired.

Locate an Exercise Partner: Assign yourself to an accountability partner or workout buddy who has like objectives and who can offer companionship, encouragement, and support. The trip can become more joyful and satisfying if you have someone with whom to share your accomplishments and setbacks.

8. Accept the Process:

Put Your Attention on advancement, Not Perfection: Accept the fact that advancement isn't always straight forward and welcome the opportunity for development. Remain dedicated to your long-term goal, acknowledge minor accomplishments, and draw lessons from failures.

Savor the Journey: Rather than concentrating only on the destination, find happiness and contentment in the process of getting there. Accept the journey of self-improvement, self-mastery, and self-discovery, and relish the sense of accomplishment that comes from fervently and purposefully pursuing your fitness objectives.

Tracking your progress, acknowledging your accomplishments, remaining adaptable, and establishing new goals will help you keep up the momentum and advance on your fitness journey. Keep in mind that creating and modifying goals are continuous processes, and being flexible and strong will help you get through any bumps in the road. You will succeed when you put in the necessary effort, perseverance, and positive thinking to keep going forward.

## Creating a Community of Support for Fitness

Creating a positive fitness community can improve your motivation, overall health, and experience with exercise tremendously. A community offers support, accountability, and companionship, which enhances the enjoyment and sustainability of the journey toward fitness objectives. The following are some ideas for developing a motivating fitness community:

1. Find People Who Share Your Thoughts:

Join Exercise Groups or Classes: Get involved in local running clubs, sports leagues, or group exercise classes. Having people around you who have similar interests and fitness objectives can help you feel connected and at home.

Connect Online: Participate in social media groups, forums, and online fitness communities that are centered around your desired objectives or activities. These platforms offer chances to interact with people from different places and backgrounds, exchange experiences, and ask for advice.

2. Encourage Good Connections:

Be Helpful: Give your fellow community members support, inspiration, and encouragement. Honor their accomplishments, provide support during trying times, and serve as an inspiration and source of optimism.

Engage in Active Listening and Empathy: When engaging with members of your fitness community, demonstrate these skills. Acknowledge their experiences, lend a sympathetic ear, and offer unprejudiced, compassionate support.

3. Plan Group Exercises:

Plan Exercises Together: Get members of your fitness community to join you on bike rides, hikes, or group workouts. Joining up for exercise together fosters friendship, support, and shared experiences.

Take Part in Challenges: Encourage the people in your community to take part in fitness challenges, like virtual races, step challenges, or fitness competitions. These exercises encourage teamwork and healthy competition while keeping everyone active.

## 4. Distribute Information and Resources:

Exchange Advice and Tips: Let other members of your fitness community benefit from your knowledge, encounters, and resources. To assist one another on their fitness journeys, give each other pointers, counsel, and suggestions on exercises, diet, equipment, and recuperation techniques.

Learn from One Another: Remain receptive to acquiring knowledge from fellow community members who possess varying perspectives, levels of expertise, or life experiences. Accept diversity and inclusiveness in your community and value the perspectives and backgrounds of all people.

5. Honor accomplishments and landmarks:

Recognize Progress: Within your fitness community, acknowledge and celebrate milestones, successes, and accomplishments of all sizes. Acknowledge accomplishments such as personal bests, fitness benchmarks, and growth spurts, and support one another along the journey.

Establish a Supportive Culture: Encourage your fitness community to be positive, encouraging, and inclusive. Establish a warm, inviting environment where everyone feels appreciated, encouraged, and free to pursue their fitness objectives.

6. Maintain Contact:

Maintain Regular Communication: Whether it's through online forums, virtual get-togethers, or in-person meetups, stay in touch with your fitness community by maintaining regular communication channels. Update each other on achievements, discuss difficulties, and provide constant encouragement and support.

Celebrate with Us: As a community, we should commemorate important days, occasions, and accomplishments. Throw get-togethers, potlucks, or parties with a fitness theme to create deeper connections and stronger ties outside of the gym.

7. Set an example for others to follow:

Set an example for others to follow by modeling the attitudes and conduct you want to see in the fitness community. Encourage others to follow your example by showcasing your commitment, tenacity, and optimism throughout your personal fitness journey.

Encourage Participation: Motivate everyone in your fitness community to actively participate and engage. Make it possible for everyone to participate, to express their distinct viewpoints, and to play a crucial role in the development and prosperity of the community.

You can build a network of like-minded people who encourage and support one another on their fitness journeys by fostering a positive fitness community. As a team, you can conquer obstacles, recognize successes, and enjoy the satisfaction that comes with working toward overall wellness and health.

## Workout Outside the Gym

There is much more to fitness than only working out at a traditional gym. Beyond the gym, there are plenty of other opportunities to maintain an active and healthy lifestyle, even if clubs offer great equipment and resources for working out. The following are some suggestions for integrating fitness outside of the gym into your everyday life:

1. Outdoor Activities: Hiking: For beautiful hikes that combine exercise with a sense of connection to nature, check out the parks and trails in your area.

Cycling: To get some exercise and fresh air, ride your bike in your neighborhood, on designated bike paths, or on beautiful routes.

Swimming: Make use of the lakes, beaches, and pools in your area for relaxing swims that train your entire body.

2. Functional Fitness: Exercises Using Your Bodyweight Exercise using your own body weight by doing push-ups, squats, lunges, and planks at home or in parks or playgrounds.

Resistance Bands: As a portable workout option, resistance bands can be used for strength training exercises that target different muscle areas.

Suspension Training: A variety of bodyweight workouts that test stability and core strength can be performed with suspension trainers such as TRX.

3. Group Exercise: Outdoor Classes: Take part in outdoor exercise programs like yoga, boot camps, or circuit training sessions at nearby parks or outdoor spaces.

Participate in community sports such as soccer, basketball, volleyball, or ultimate frisbee by joining recreational teams or leagues.

Dance Classes: Attend Zumba, salsa, or hip-hop classes in parks or community centers.

4. Active Transportation: Walking: Whenever practical, walk to work, school, or run errands as part of your daily routine.

Cycling: For errands around town or as a means of transportation, use a bicycle.

Public Transit: To increase daily steps and physical activity, get off the bus or train one or two stations early and walk the entire distance.

5. Online Workouts: Workouts at Home Get access to streaming services or online fitness programs to do guided workouts from the comfort of your home.

Fitness Apps: Get fitness apps with features like exercise demos, individualized training plans, and progress monitoring.

Equipment for the Home: For easy workouts at home, get yourself some dumbbells, kettlebells, yoga mats, or stability balls.

6. Active Recreation: Gardening: Take part in physically active and stress-relieving gardening tasks like planting, weeding, digging, and watering.

Take on physical labor-intensive DIY projects around the house, like painting, carpentry, or landscaping.

Recreational Sports: For an entertaining and active way to pass the time, try your hand at recreational sports and activities like rock climbing, tennis, golf, or kayaking.

7. Social and Family Activities: Going on family bike rides or walks is a great way to strengthen relationships and keep the family active.

Playtime with Pets: Take your pets on active playdates, including fetch games, jogs, or hikes through the outdoors.

Social Events: Plan fun get-togethers with friends and family, such picnics, beach outings, or outdoor sports like soccer or frisbee.

8. Mind-Body Techniques: Outdoor Meditation or Yoga Take a yoga or meditation class outside in peaceful natural environments, such as gardens, parks, or beaches.

Qigong or Tai Chi: For moderate movement, relaxation, and stress relief, learn and practice Qigong or Tai Chi outside.

Walking with awareness: When you stroll in the outdoors, walk with awareness of your surroundings, your breathing, and your body's sensations.

You can take advantage of a wide variety of physical activities that meet your interests, lifestyle, and surroundings by embracing fitness outside of the gym. There are several ways to make health and well-being a priority in your daily life, whether you're remaining active at home, going on outdoor adventures, or attending group exercise programs. Try a variety of things, discover what makes you happy, and incorporate movement into your daily routine to maintain your long-term health and vigor.

## Overcoming Typical Obstacles in Fitness

Reaching your health and wellness objectives and keeping up a regular workout regimen depend on conquering typical fitness obstacles. Even though there can be roadblocks along the way, there are tactics you can use to get beyond them and continue on your fitness path. Here are some typical obstacles to fitness and how to get past them:

1. Lack of motivation:

Establish Specific Objectives: Establish attainable, measurable fitness objectives that will drive and excite you. Having specific goals gives your workouts direction and purpose, whether it's increasing flexibility, lifting a certain amount of weight, or running a specific distance.

Discover Your Motive: Think about the motivations behind your desire to make fitness a priority in your life. Rekindling your love for exercise might come from reconnecting with your underlying motivations, whether they are to improve health, increase energy, manage stress, or improve performance in a particular activity.

Mix It Up: Try a variety of exercises, events, and classes to keep your training interesting and unique. To avoid boredom, try out other sports, outdoor activities, or training regimens.

2. Time Limitations:

Make exercise a priority: Workouts should be scheduled as non-negotiable appointments in your daily schedule. Set aside time each day for physical activity, treating it like any other significant obligation.

Optimize Efficiency: Choose workouts that will yield the most advantages in the shortest amount of time. When time is of the essence, high-intensity interval training (HIIT), circuit training, and Tabata workouts are great ways to fit in a short and efficient workout.

Split It Up: If planning a lengthy workout seems unattainable, break it up into smaller, more manageable sessions spread out throughout the day. Over time, even brief active intervals can have a major positive impact on your health.

3. Inconsistency: Begin Little: As you gain confidence and endurance, start with small goals and progressively increase the intensity, length, and frequency. Make an effort to develop dependable routines and habits that you can stick with in the long run.

Establish Accountability: Look for a coach, exercise partner, or accountability partner who can assist you in staying on track with your fitness objectives. Having a support system, someone to check in with, and someone to discuss success with helps boost motivation and accountability.

Track Your Progress: To keep yourself accountable for your workouts and goals, keep a workout journal, utilize a fitness app, or wear a fitness tracker. Exercise logs, accomplishment journals, and milestone celebrations all support the preservation of motivation and momentum.

4. Unexpected Outcomes: Establish Reasonable Expectations When it comes to your fitness quest, remember that development requires

patience and consistency—be realistic and patient. Instead of comparing yourself to other people, concentrate on developing yourself.

Assess Your Approach: To find areas for improvement, assess your exercise regimen, eating habits, sleep hygiene, and stress-reduction strategies. Seek advice and support from a nutritionist or fitness expert for individualized advice.

Celebrate Non-Scale Victories: Disregard the scale and give attention to non-scale achievements like heightened strength, enhanced endurance, better sleep, and improved happiness. Acknowledge and rejoice in every positive transformation exercise makes in your life, not just the physical one.

5. Injury Risk: Give Safety First Priority: When exercising, pay attention to your body's needs and put safety first by employing the right form, technique, and equipment. To avoid overuse injuries, begin gradually, warm up appropriately, and use rest days and recovery procedures.

Cross-Train: To avoid overuse injuries and balance muscle development, mix up your program by incorporating different workouts and activities. In addition to offering cerebral stimulation, cross-training lowers the chance of burnout.

Seek Professional Advice: Consult a certified fitness professional, such as a personal trainer or physical therapist, if you have questions regarding appropriate form, technique, or exercise choices. They can evaluate your movement patterns, offer tailored advice, and assist in avoiding injuries.

6. Mental Difficulties:

Exercise Self-Compassion: Recognize that obstacles and disappointments are a normal part of the fitness path and treat yourself with kindness. Develop resilience, self-compassion, and an optimistic outlook to get beyond mental obstacles and maintain motivation.

Attend to Mental Health Needs: See a mental health expert for assistance if mental health conditions like stress, anxiety, or depression are impairing your motivation and general wellbeing. Underlying mental obstacles to fitness can be addressed with the aid of therapy, counseling, or stress-reduction methods.

Discover Joy in Movement: Pay attention to pursuits and workouts that make you happy, fulfilled, and proud of yourself. Pick physical activities that you enjoy doing, such as dancing, hiking, swimming, or sports. This will make working out more fun.

7. Adapt to Change in the Environment: When faced with environmental obstacles like bad weather, travel, or restricted access to facilities, exercise flexibility and adaptability. Accept the challenge of coming up with inventive ideas, adapt exercises as necessary, and look for different methods to be active no matter what.

Exercise at Home: Set up a small exercise area in your house with a yoga mat, resistance bands, and dumbbells as your only equipment. For quick and efficient at-home workouts, use fitness applications, virtual training sessions, or online workout videos.

Outdoor Options: Use open fields, parks, and trails as locations for outdoor exercises and recreation. Explore the great outdoors for sunshine, fresh air, and breathtaking views. Use nature as your gym.

You may overcome hurdles, stick to your fitness objectives, and eventually achieve increased health and well-being by identifying and resolving common fitness issues with proactive techniques and a positive mindset. Recall that development may not always follow a straight line and that obstacles present chances for improvement. You may overcome obstacles and integrate exercise into a fulfilling and long-lasting aspect of your lifestyle if you have perseverance, determination, and the flexibility to change.

## Motivation and Assistance for Readers

To every reader starting a fitness journey:

I would want to take this opportunity to thank you for your dedication to putting your health and wellbeing first via your pursuit of fitness. Whether you're a beginner, a seasoned athlete making a comeback, or a self-imposed challenger, know that every step you take toward your fitness objectives is an accomplishment worthy of celebration.

It's acceptable to face obstacles along the way because the road to fitness is not always straightforward. As a matter of fact, conquering challenges is a natural part of the process and enhances your mental and physical toughness. Recall that progress is sometimes determined by the number on the scale or the distance traveled; sometimes, it's about the experience, the development, and the changes you go through on the route.

I want you to embrace patience and persistence, treat yourself with kindness, and recognize and appreciate every small triumph along your fitness journey. Every accomplishment, be it finishing a difficult workout, breaking through a mental barrier, or just getting out of bed every morning, is a tribute to your fortitude, resiliency, and commitment.

Recognize that you are not traveling alone. Seek out assistance from loved ones, friends, or other fitness enthusiasts who can motivate and inspire you as you progress. Talk to others about your achievements, struggles, and goals; you can also gain inspiration from their journeys.

Above all, keep in mind that being fit involves more than just working out physically; it also involves taking care of your body, mind, and spirit in order to create a lifetime of vitality, health, and well-being. Accept the pleasure of activity, the thrill of advancement, and the sense of power that comes from managing your health.

Remember that you are capable, deserving, and entitled to all the advantages that fitness has to offer, regardless of where you are in your fitness journey. Continue to believe in yourself, keep moving forward, and continue to show up. Your path is distinct, and there are countless options.

I'm wishing you courage, resiliency, and unending success in your journey to fitness.

## CONCLUSION

In summary, achieving fitness is a holistic process that involves self-evolution, empowerment, and self-discovery in addition to physical change. We've covered a wide range of the effects that exercise has on our lives in this book, from strengthening and promoting physical health to boosting resilience and mental health.

We've covered topics including how to overcome typical obstacles, enjoy the process of moving, and create a network of allies that can encourage and uplift us while traveling. We've acknowledged the abundance of fitness options available, both inside and outside of the gym, and we've pushed one another to accept the journey with tolerance, persistence, and self-compassion.

By the time this book ends, I hope you will be inspired, uplifted, and prepared to tackle your next fitness challenge with renewed vigor and determination. Recall that physical activity is a lifelong quest of health, energy, and wellbeing rather than a destination. Every action, decision, and challenge you encounter advances your physical, mental, and spiritual well-being and brings you one step closer to your objectives.

I want to urge you to stay true to yourself, pay attention to your body, and prioritize self-care and balance as you move forward on your fitness journey. Reward yourself for your successes, take lessons from your failures, and never stop challenging yourself. And never forget that you deserve a life full of happiness, joy, and health since you are strong, robust, and capable.

I appreciate you going on this journey with me. May you have strength, happiness, and an endless amount of opportunities ahead of you.

# THE END